BREAKING THE SILENCE: DEATH OF A SUPERWOMAN

MY EXPERIENCE WITH SJOGRENS SYNDROME AND CHRONIC ILLNESS

Copyright©2015 by Ayanna Henry.

For my two greatest heroes, my mom and my uncle. You know why.

For T. Harbin, for planting the seed.

For D. Polk, for believing it would grow.

Acknowledgments

Wow! I cannot believe this project is finally completed! I would like to thank and acknowledge the following special people for their assistance, input, and guidance:

Thank you, God, for your many blessings and for the inspiration to begin this book!

My mother and my brothers, who have always been there for me and with me and keep me continually grounded.

My niece, Amina McCrary (my mini-me), for being one of the first to read one of my drafts and for your constant presence in my life. You are truly heaven sent!

My oldest and dearest friend, Arlean J. Worthy, who I have known since she was 4 and I was 6 (smile), thank you for allowing me to share my private world with you and for you sharing your private world with me! (We are more than conquerors!)

My bestie, Angela Smith, who remains by my side through it all, my love for you is beyond words.

And to the following friends, family and former co-workers who I enlisted to read my early drafts and gave me the courage to move forward anyway: Leisa Simms-Thomas, Celestine Huntley, Veronica Berry, Coryus Veal, Tarcella Jones, Traveese Harbin, Danny Polk, Sonja McCray, and Verona Davis.

My good friend and confidante, Richard Wright, who has supported me from Day 1 and continues to uplift me.

And to anyone else that has assisted me in any way, whether through an encouraging word on a bad day, to actually reading my story and giving me feedback, if I forgot to list your name, count it to my head and not to my heart.

Thank you all so much! Much love!

Well, I am finally beginning to write the book that I have been told by many that I should have written.

I thought that when I finally began to write a book that it would be about my life experiences.

But the universe had a different plan.

This book will be the story of my life but it will also be about my death.

Not death in the physical sense, of course, because, obviously I am still here typing.

But the death of a superwoman.

Or someone who thought she was……

I am the type of person that has always had to have her back against the wall before I would do what I needed to do for myself.

I was good at getting things done at work, at home, and for others.

But I failed miserably in taking care of myself.

And it almost cost me my life. The very illnesses that I thought would kill me actually saved me.

For if I continued on the course that I was taking, I believe that I would have surely died or lost my mind.

It took several bouts of chronic illness to begin to wake me up from my selfimposed sleep.

It would be the diagnosis and experience with an unknown disease that would propel me into action.

This is my story. I endured pain and suffering alone for many years because I did not want to burden others with my problems.

But I have recently discovered that I cannot heal until I release.

So, it is my hope that in breaking my silence that it will help someone else.

Maybe even save their life as mine was saved.

This book will be a little unique and unusual as it will not be organized as a traditional story would be.

I have recorded my experiences in my journal writings over the past several years, so instead of retelling and recalling the events from my memory, I will invite you into my private thoughts during my day to day experiences.

Enter at your own risk.

I wasn't sure how to begin my story. Some people would say, "Just start from the beginning", but I'm not so sure where that beginning is anymore, so I will just start from now.

Today is April 1, 2013. I am 41 years old. I never imagined I would live to this age, nor be present in this time of life. But I am. And lived to tell about it.

I am currently at home on leave from work. Medical leave. I was diagnosed last year with a disease called Sjogren's Syndrome. **SJOGRENS** (pronounced Showgrins). I know, nothing like it sounds. Sjogrens Syndrome is an autoimmune disease similar to Lupus that attacks the body's exocrine or moisture producing glands. It is primarily characterized by dry eyes and dry mouth, however, it can also affect many other parts of the body as well as major organs.

I have experienced just about the full gamut of the disease so I decided to write about my experience in my own words. I have read several books and case studies online about other people's experiences with the disease, so I figured I might as well share mine.

This all began just after was finishing up my Master's degree in 2011. I was determined to finish prior to my 40th birthday, which was in January of 2012. Everything was proceeding on schedule until the fall of 2011. I had been having pain in my right hand, off and on, I felt it especially while I was driving. I started pressing it all over to see what the source of the pain was and I found a pea size nodule below my middle finger. It was tender to the touch and was mobile within my hand. After trying to ignore it for some time, I finally decided to visit my primary care doctor, Dr. D. He referred me to a hand specialist, Dr. G. After being examined by Dr. G, I was told I had a benign ganglion cyst in my hand that needed to be surgically removed.

The surgery date was set for November 3, 2011 (Unfortunately, this was also Lyric's 2nd birthday, Lyric is my goddaughter, so I missed her birthday because I was at the hospital). In addition to that, I was scheduled for midterms that same week. I had no choice, last class, last semester. The last class was my final Tax law course, dealing with Taxation of Non-Profit organizations.

I had the surgery done, outpatient. It went as planned, just felt woozy after, and I vomited on the way home. The surgery was done on Thursday, November 3, and on the next day, Friday, I had to take part one of the midterm. My brother, Atiba, was so gracious to do the honors of escorting the patient to Nova, since I could not drive.

I was still an utter mess on Friday, but I went to class with my sling, brace and all and completed the first part of the exam. Saturday morning, the next day,

Atiba returned me to Nova to complete the remainder of the exam. My Tax Law instructor asked me if I had been in a fight since I showed up with a sling. He wanted to know what the other person looked like.

I passed my exams and completed the requirements for my Master's Degree. It should have been a happy time, right? Wrong! Right after I recovered from the hand surgery, I came down with a bad cold and then had a weird infection in my scalp.

Dr. "D", my primary doctor, didn't seem to take it too seriously, but I literally had boils in my head that burned really bad.

I next went to Dr. T, another doctor in Dr. D's office and was given 3 types of antibiotics (Amoxicillin, Cipro, and a strong dose of another one I cannot recall, it was like 850 mg). Immediately after that I developed a dry and hacking cough that lingered over 2 months. I went back to the doctor and was given an inhaler and also advised that possibly excess acid was producing the mucus. I didn't believe any of it. I had next developed a very bad earache on the left side, went back to the doctor and was given ear drops for that. I now had an ear infection. I never get those! Finally, in February of 2012, still not having found any relief from the meds I had been given, I put myself on a regimen of herbs,

Echinacea and Golden Seal, for about 2 weeks and then noticed some improvement.

After that episode calmed down, new things started to pop up in March 2012. I began to experience blurred vision, sensitivity to light, joint pain and pain all over my body. I felt like my body was shutting down. So I took myself back to Dr. D in mid-March to assess the problem. What was happening to me? I could barely drive there, my feet hurt so badly that I could not touch the pedals without being in pain.

I explained all of my symptoms to Dr. D who immediately performed a thorough exam and a complete battery of lab tests and X-Rays to see if he could find the cause.

The lab work included a rheumatoid profile, with tests for Lupus, Rheumatoid Arthritis, etc. This was important since I have a genetic predisposition for autoimmune diseases. My mother has had Lupus, Fibromyalgia, and Rheumatoid Arthritis for over 20 years and is currently on disability. My uncle has had Multiple Sclerosis for almost 20 years and is also currently on disability and has lost most of his ability to walk.

What I did not know at the time is that the lab work also included a test for a disease called Sjogren's. I had no clue what was wrong with me, but I knew it was not all in my head.

I received a call from Dr. D within a few days with results of the tests.

He told me the tests were positive for Sjogren's and also showed high levels of inflammation in my body. I didn't know the first thing about this strangely named disease nor how I was to handle receiving this news.

Meanwhile, my health continued to deteriorate greatly. My eyes could not tolerate any type of bright light/sunlight, and I had extreme episodes of fatigue and burning pain of my hands and feet. I had a headache for the last few days that I couldn't get rid of. I have been taking the Neurontin, Ibuprofen, and as a last resort, Vicodin to manage the pain. I have been using my heating pad for the pain in my back.

So many things were going on that I had no explanation for. At least I had the presence of mind to recognize that I could no longer continue working in this state, so I had already informed my Supervisor of my deteriorating condition even before I received a diagnosis and had my doctor complete the necessary paperwork to place me on extended sick leave as of the end of March.

I was then referred to a rheumatologist, either Dr. K, my mother's long time rheumatologist, or I could find one on my own. I was fortunate enough to find

Dr. P., a rheumatologist in the Bennett Medical Building where most of my other doctors were. I needed to get in to see her as soon as possible so that I could get some help.

I couldn't get an appointment for Dr. P until the middle of April, which means I had to suffer for at least another 2-3 weeks before I could receive any sort of treatment or medication.

When my appointment date finally came, I found Dr. P" to be kind, compassionate, and thorough.

She felt that my condition was a combination of the Sjogren's and Fibromyalgia.

She started me on Prednisone steroids and told me I had to wait to be placed on the Plaquenil that is the drug of choice for treatment of Sjogren's. I needed to be cleared by an ophthalmologist before I could begin taking the Plaquenil. I began taking the Plaquenil in May 2012.

There have been many ups and downs since. Burning eyes, no tears. Oh yeah, if I try to cry it burns something awful and nothing happens. Maybe a trickle or two of water, but nothing else.

I guess that's God's way of telling me He doesn't want me to cry anymore, because I have certainly shed my share of tears in this life.

Clogged nasal passages, dry mouth, recurrent diarrhea (you don't really want to know), burning pain in my hands and feet, and the worst fatigue ever. I have episodes where I get really tired and can pass out asleep without warning. Sometimes it lasts a few minutes or a few hours.

Then it takes time to snap out of it.

So that was how it all began. Flash forward back to the present day.

Since this ordeal began last year, I have been in and out of work.

I might have a good few weeks then I have to call out sick. I might be out a few days at its best or a few weeks or longer at its worst.

Sjogrens has a mind of its own and I have no control over it whatsoever. It is totally unpredictable. I never know how I am going to feel. I wake up one day with energy and take a bath and just that quickly the energy is gone.

So here I am. Dealing with this Sjogrens. What does this all mean?

That's what I've been trying to figure out. What is it? Why did this happen to all of us? My mom? My uncle? And now me?

And what do I do now?

I often find myself wondering when my problems with illness and my health began. As I look back in time, I believe this whole ordeal began in 1993.

I was 21 years old and working full time at the Boys and Girls Clubs of Broward County.

I worked crazy hours as the Administrative Coordinator to the Director of Operations. 12, 14, and 16 hour days along with 7 day work weeks were pretty much the norm for me.

I lived with my boyfriend at the time, but I barely saw him because I was always working.

Sometime during that year, I caught a very bad cold that took over a month to get over. This was no ordinary cold, either. I had nausea, vomiting, and diarrhea along with chills and fever. I didn't know if it was a cold, flu, or something else more serious. I just wanted to feel better. I was constantly in the bathroom either vomiting or it was coming out the other way. My boyfriend, to his credit, was forced to take care of me, since I could not do anything for myself.

I saw my doctor and was given antibiotics, which I did not respond to.

I found myself getting sicker and increasingly more tired each day. My mom, who was diagnosed with

Lupus and Chronic Fatigue Syndrome a few years prior, saw my plight and based on her own experience, thought there might be something more than a cold going on with me, so she wanted to take me to the Cleveland Clinic. "I'm sure they will find the problem", she told me.

So on to the Cleveland Clinic we went. The doctor there ran a battery of tests, bloodwork, etc. But the only thing conclusive the tests showed were high levels of the Epstein-Barr virus, the virus that is predominately linked to Chronic Fatigue Syndrome or CFIDs and Mononucleosis.

I was told by the doctor that I most likely have CFIDs based on the blood tests and my symptoms. I was sent home and placed on extended bed rest. I was not given any medication or treatment at that time.

I was forced to leave my job temporarily and remain at home to rest and recover, which I finally did after a few months. I then returned to college to continue working toward my degree.

The CFIDs? Or whatever I had did not resurface again until 2001.

It should really be no surprise since I was back to my workaholic/superwoman ways again.

I was now working in the Human Resources Department. Back to working 12, 14, and 16 hour days as well as weekends. I even started taking work home with me. I had to, because our agency served over 6000 employees at the time, during the day I was constantly on the phone, sending emails and seeing employees at the front counter. It was nearly impossible to keep up with my workload, so myself and others in my department often stayed after hours to complete our work.

I was also taking a few classes at the university, continuing to work towards my Bachelor's degree. All of this while attempting to run my house, take my mom to her doctor's appointments, and whatever else came up.

It all became too much for me. I was burning out, but I didn't know how to stop myself.

When I was about to lose hope, I saw a job opening as a secretary at the Chaplain's Office. The hours were 9 to 5, but it was a more stable work environment, and more than likely I would be home at a reasonable time each day and have my weekends to myself again.

This should be a great place to work, I thought to myself. It's the "Chaplain's Office", for crying out loud!

So I applied for the position and I got the job!

Things started out fine in the beginning. I was much more at ease and in a relaxed atmosphere, but my body was still feeling the effects of working all of those hours in Human Resources.

I didn't want to admit it, but I was slowly breaking down. In spite of changing jobs, I was totally exhausted all of the time and began to have flu-like symptoms, such as chills and fever. I also kept a sore throat. This along with body aches and fatigue began to overwhelm me.

I finally reached the breaking point and totally fell apart.

My primary doctor sent me to a rheumatologist after lab tests again indicated high levels of the Epstein-Barr virus.

I was formally diagnosed with Chronic Fatigue Syndrome (CFIDS). Here we go again!

The rheumatologist I went to was my mother's long time rheumatologist, Dr. K. He confirmed the diagnosis of CFIDs, but because my mom, who has Lupus, is also his patient, he advised me that at some point in the future I would more than likely develop an autoimmune disease. It may be Lupus, or something else, but based on my current condition, the likelihood is high.

Dr. K. prescribed Elavil for the pain. This began a cycle of me going from my primary doctor to the rheumatologist and then to a neurologist in order to manage my care. I was subsequently placed on Paxil, Zoloft, Prozac, Neurontin, Xanax, and a strange drug called Pamelor or Nortriptyline. I was also on medication for the bad migraines I suddenly developed.

None of these drugs had any lasting benefit, with the exception of the Neurontin. The Elavil and Nortriptyline make me feel like a walking zombie.

The others had no effect at all, so I stopped taking all but the Neurontin.

I was back to square one and barely making it to work each day.

My work hours were 830 am – 500 p.m., Monday-Friday. I was not arriving at work most days until 10 or 1030 am. Thankfully the Chaplain was compassionate and worked with me, allowing me to adjust my hours to 10 to 6, or whatever time I came in, I worked an 8 hour day from then.

Then there were the days I didn't show up at all. Many times I would get up and attempt to get dressed, and be so exhausted I couldn't make it out of the house.

I was struggling with excessive daytime fatigue because I had difficulty sleeping at night due to aches and pains. I was placed on light duty for a while by my primary doctor, and limited to a 30 hour work week to see if my symptoms improved, but to no avail.

Finally, I decided it was time to leave and try to find a job on the night shift. I figured since I couldn't sleep anyway, that would help my body get the rest it needed if I could work at night and sleep during the day.

So I began to pray for a job opening in another department that had shift work. To my surprise and relief, my prayers were quickly answered.

I saw an opening in my former department, the Warrants Division. This was my very first job with the agency, and I had left there 2 years prior to accept a promotion to the position in Human Resources.

I phoned my previous supervisor in Warrants to inquire about the hours for the opening. I needed to ensure there would be a night shift available or it wouldn't be worth it to apply. She said the opening was indeed for the night shift and I told her I was interested, and she replied that they would hire me back in a heartbeat.

Long story short, I applied for and got the job in Warrants and returned to Warrants in May of 2002. After working the night shift for several months, thankfully my health began to improve. I loved the hours! Eventually, I began to feel like my former self. I remained there for the next 4 years, fluctuating between the 11 p.m. to 7 a.m. shift and the 3 p.m. to 11 p.m. shift. Those later shifts seemed to agree with me better.

Thyroid Disease/Hashimoto's Thyroiditis/Total Thyroidectomy

2006 -2009

In August of 2006, I graduated from Florida Atlantic University with a Bachelor of Business Administration in Finance.

This was no small feat as I had to work full time while going to school as well as support my family.

It took me 14 years to complete this task from the time I received my Associates Degree in 1992.

I was completely exhausted when I finished as well as relieved when it was all over. I was also looking forward to moving on with my life and to a new career, right? Wrong.

I figured it would take several months to a year before I fully recovered from the stress of all those late nights writing papers and preparing for presentations. In addition, I started a new job in June of 2006, just before graduation.

But the fatigue and exhaustion continued to linger well into 2007. I began to wonder just what was going on with me.

I also noticed a gradual weight gain, so subtle that I almost didn't notice it until I couldn't fit my clothes anymore.

By August of 2007, one year following graduation, I had gained almost 40 pounds.

On top of that, I developed a sore throat that also lingered for over a year.

Now I knew something was wrong.

I had been seeing my primary doctor periodically during this time and advising him of the sore throat and fatigue. He thought that these might be by products of the stress of finishing school.

He suggested rest would resolve them.

But it did not. So back to him I went.

This time he ordered lab tests to check my thyroid levels (since my mom had a thyroid problem, I may also), but the tests were normal.

My health continued to decline and I continued to work throughout.

I was always tired, weary, and sluggish.

And I had still had that unexplained sore throat along with a feeling like I had hair caught in the back in my throat (this constantly made me feel like I had to gag).

Finally, I had reached my limit and demanded to see a specialist in the fall of 2007. "If they don't find anything, then I'll let it go", I told my primary.

So off to Dr. M. I went (Ear/Nose/Throat doctor). He performed several examinations that included looking at the inside of my throat with a camera.

Dr. M. advised that my thyroid was enlarged and recommended that I have an ultrasound of the thyroid done to take a closer look.

I had the ultrasound completed and the results showed a tumor (mass) on the left side of my neck and several nodules on the right. Things moved fairly quickly after that.

I was then sent to an endocrinologist to be further evaluated and to determine the future course of action.

The endocrinologist sent me for a fine needle biopsy to examine the tissue of thyroid to check for any malignancies.

Once done, we could move forward from there.

The biopsy was "suspicious for malignancy", and my endocrinologist was not taking any chances – I was told I had to have surgery as soon as possible to remove the entire thyroid, a total thyroidectomy.

Within the next few months and several more tests and doctor visits, I was scheduled for surgery in March 2008, and again in June of 2008(my thyroidectomy was done in 2 parts, much to the chagrin of my endocrinologist).

They found cancer in the tumor itself, but since it was contained within the tumor, once the thyroid was removed, the cancer was as well.

Thankfully, I did not require any radiation or chemotherapy treatments, but I was placed on Synthroid or thyroid replacement hormone, which takes the place of the absent thyroid gland, and which I will be required to take for the rest of my life.

I will also need to be monitored by an endocrinologist for the rest of my life with lab work every few months and an annual thyroid ultrasound.

I will gladly submit to these things since I was spared from radiation and chemotherapy.

Now back to the Sjogren's experience.

In the beginning stages of the disease, the dry mouth was so severe that I could barely chew or swallow. I frequently awakened to my lips being stuck together. My tongue and the inside of my mouth were so inflamed and burning that I was forced to seek medical attention and was told I had an infection – oral thrush, that was treated by Dr. M.

I suffered from frequent diarrhea several times a week, and I did not receive any relief until I was finally sent to a gastroenterologist for assistance. I had a colonoscopy in April of 2013 that provided some relief from the diarrhea, however, it does return periodically during flares.

Also, during this period, I have been in and out of work since these symptoms were extremely debilitating and I was unable to work for more than a few days at a time, if at all. By the beginning of March 2013, I had completely exhausted my sick leave and vacation time at work.

I can be a very determined person when I want to be, also to my detriment. When I returned from sick leave in April of 2013, after my colonoscopy, I had made up my mind to push as hard as I could to work as long as I could without taking any sick leave. I was very proud of myself for going a full six months without being out sick. This is not to say that I did not take any time off, because I did, however, I did not call out sick during this time.

This was very difficult to do, and I expended most, if not all, of my energy to attempt to work and would often return home completely exhausted and depleted.

Most of my days off are spent in bed since I have no energy to do anything else, so I spend the time recuperating in order to return to work reasonably refreshed.

Have I experienced any improvement with this disease since the initial diagnosis almost 3 years ago? Yes and No. Sjogren's is a very unpredictable disease. I can wake up in the morning feeling well, and 2 hours later, feel like the wind was knocked out of me. Or, sometimes, a particular activity, for example, taking a shower or bath, can totally exhaust me.

A flare can occur without warning, and I never know how long it is going to last. They have lasted from 20 minutes to 2 weeks, or longer. They have varied from mild to unbearable. When flare occurs, I have to take immediate rest or at least cease all activity as soon as possible. If I do not, it gets progressively worse.

What happens during a flare

The first telltale signs of a flare for me are the burning eyes and light sensitivity. My eyes are so sensitive at this time that I cannot even look at my television screen, as the light emanating from the TV is too bright. My room is already kept as dark as possible because I keep the blinds closed during the day. In extreme cases, I have actually lied in bed with the blankets over my head because I could not take any light at all. I keep my lamp and overhead lights off most of the time as well. I have been forced to purchase polarized eye glass lenses and have had the Transitions lenses that automatically adjust to the light applied to my regular frames.

The burning eyes usually occur after a stressful event or too much activity. How much activity is too much? Sometimes I can clean the bathroom and that is too much. I can sweep the floor in my room, and that is too much. Whatever the trigger, when the eyes start burning, it is generally the first sign that I need to stop.

Next, the fatigue and pain begin. I become extremely tired, not in the ordinary sense, but fatigued to the point where I feel completely drained and devoid of energy. I have slept for days at a time in the early stages of the disease. And usually have to lay down and rest when at this point. I also have the burning, tingling, and numbness of my hands and feet. This is a highly painful sensation. I feel like my hands and especially my feet are on fire. It has literally brought tears to my eyes. I can barely walk during this time.

It has also been causing problems with my driving. Sometimes I cannot feel the accelerator pedal under my feet. I have difficulty with sensation at the bottom of my feet, particularly the right foot.

I am barely making it to work and I am beginning to lose my willpower. Every week lately I am ready to give up. I am no longer feeling like it is worth it for me to continue to push on any longer. I usually keep all of my feelings inside, but I cannot remain silent any longer.

Generally, I try to maintain a positive attitude most of the time, even when I am not feeling well, because I have always been the type of person not to complain, even to my own detriment. And I also have the tendency to wait until a medical issue has become unbearable before I have sought medical attention.

Unfortunately, this habit of mine leads one to believe that I am not as physically ill as I really am. I am literally struggling to get to work every day.

The below is a list of symptoms that I have endured since I was diagnosed with this disease in 2012:

    Burning Eyes/Dry Eyes/Blurred Vision

    Sensitivity to Light

- Dry Mouth
- Frequent/Recurrent Sinus Problems
- Extreme Fatigue
- Nerve Pain/Burning /Tingling of Hands and Feet
- Oral Thrush
- Diarrhea
- Body Aches/Joint/Muscle Aches
- Nausea
- Sore Throat/Dry Cough
- Reflux
- Dizziness
- Difficulty Concentrating (Brain Fog)

These symptoms wax and wane during "flares". I have been experiencing several flares a week since this all began.

I have been to the following specialists for treatment of the disease:

- Rheumatologist

Neurologist

Ophthalmologist

Gastroenterologist

Pulmonologist

Ear/Nose/Throat/Specialist

Dentist

Here are a few of my journal entries that outlines my experience:

8/7/14

I am currently at home again on sick leave for possibly the next 3 months. I have been having a bad flare since the end of June.

I fought it as long as I could, but reached the point where I could no longer fight and had to lay my sword down and stay home and rest.

My rheumatologist did all she could to try to assist with stopping the flare, she increased my Prednisone to up to 60 milligrams and also increased the Cell Cept to 2000 milligrams in an attempt to suppress the disease.

Unfortunately, the combination of the flare and the sudden increase in medications made things worse. I began to have stomach pain and nausea in addition to the fatigue, and the usual burning pain in my hands and feet.

I have been home for almost 3 weeks now, and I am just beginning to feel like myself again. The first two weeks were spent in bed, literally. I only got up to use the bathroom and every now and then, for food or drink. There were a few days that I'm not even sure if I took a bath. I was just in darkness, or, as I have described to a few friends that inquired on my wellbeing, I was "underwater".

I am at home in exile. I left the jail at work for a jail at home. I am finally beginning to feel the mental and emotional impact of suffering with this disease.

Currently, I believe I am still in some form of denial. Since I had been able to continue working for 30-60 days with minimal time off in between, I think that I felt that I was getting better, the disease was going into remission, the new meds were helping, etc.

So, I was beginning to conduct myself as if I was normal. Big mistake. Because when the flare came a calling again, I wasn't ready.

I recognized the signs, but I ignored them. I continued on like nothing was wrong and kept on pushing.

But so did he, like a lion in pursuit of his prey.

Finally, I succumbed and surrendered, mind, body, and spirit, totally spent.

I'm home and now forced to confront myself and deal with how I really feel about this illness and begin the process of making the major life changes that must happen now.

One of the hardest things for me to accept is not being able to do everything I used to do. Now there are limitations.

I have to accept that the person I used to be or thought I was, can never be again.

She has to go.

I have to accept that one day I will have to leave the jail due to my health.

I have to accept that I have a disease that has no cure.

I have to accept that I will be on all of these medications for the rest of my life.

I have to accept that I had to die so that I could live.

While being home recuperating, I was led to begin to write during my spare time away from work. So, this book is the result of my efforts.

I am a long way from becoming the new person I am to be.

I am most definitely a work in process.

I am working at coming to terms with my disease and finding a better quality of life. Being forced to sit down, and be still is the worst punishment as well as the best punishment for me.

I believe God's got jokes, He knows that sitting me down or slowing me down is the only way to get my attention and listen.

I couldn't continue going on the way that I was. All of this happened to wake me up and force me to make the changes I need to make to begin to live my life before it's too late.

I am praying for my recovery, for my restoration, and rejuvenation.

I hope that sharing my battle with Sjogren's and chronic illness in general will touch someone else who has had similar health issues and give them hope or at least comfort that they are not alone.

3/23/15

There will be no going back to work as I knew it. The last time I was out took the last bit of strength I had to fight back. I really believed when I went back last September that I would be able to stay up, to stay afloat.

With 30-50 lbs. of extra weight that I had gained from the high doses of
Prednisone that I was on, it made the journey back to work at that time extremely difficult. But I was determined to fight back, and managed to return on 9/22/14.

Unfortunately, my return was to be short lived. I fought and fought so hard to continue to go until my body shut down again in January.

So here I am at the 3rd week of March at the end of my journey. Usually, by now, I am either ready to return to work or preparing to return to work. For whatever reason, I just did not bounce back like I normally would have by now.

I'm not sure of the reason why. Maybe all of the fighting against the disease finally took its toll on my body and it just could not fight anymore.

It's difficult for me to accept this because I believed I could beat it. And I tried hard and fought with all I had!

I have thought and prayed about it and meditated and know that it is time to leave the BSO. It really has been time to leave, but my plans to leave by other means were thwarted by illness. I had intended to leave upon completing my education, whether it was my Bachelors' degree or Master's degree.

But it was not meant to be. Each time I completed a degree, I was afflicted with some disease. After the Bachelors, I found out I had a tumor in my neck and thyroid disease. After the Masters, it was Sjogren's.

I had been miserable at the job for some time now but was willing to endure it to maintain employment and my health insurance. I knew there was no future nor upward mobility but I was still grateful that I had a job and benefits.

But it seemed the more I worked and the harder I tried to get there, the worse I felt. I began to cry out to God that I was tired and couldn't go any more, do any more, take anymore. And I meant it. I told God I was willing to walk away from everything, job, house, etc., in order for things to change.

So here I am in March 2015. I did something that I never thought I would have to do this soon or at all. I submitted my application for disability retirement. My original plan was to just walk away from the job and everything else.

To resign and take whatever funds were in my pension, pay off my bills, finish fixing up the house and to go somewhere and start over.

I was determined to do just that too, but my Uncle Stevie talked me out of it and when I had a chance to think about it and to research my options, I saw that he was right. If I just resigned, I would lose my benefits, health insurance, and disability insurance.

But if I medically retired and was able to draw my short and long term disability, it would buy me some time and allow me to have some income coming in until I was able to apply for social security disability.

What I also learned is that retiring due to disability would also allow me to continue with my health insurance with a discount based on my years of service. That made the decision a little easier. So, right now at this moment, I am waiting on the last bit of paperwork from my primary doctor that needs to be submitted to the retirement system. I will be picking that up later today, 3/23/15.

The reality of all of this still has not hit me fully. Like I was explaining to my mom, I still have not gone through the separation process at the job. Cleaning out my drawer, turning in uniforms, my badge, and saying good bye.

It feels bittersweet right now. Part of me is relieved that it will be over and I have a chance to live my life differently, to pursue some things that I kept putting on a shelf for later. To learn how to love myself and care for myself properly.

But another part is terrified. This is truly venturing into the unknown. What will I do with myself? What will happen now?

I also realize that my whole life was wrapped up in the Sheriff's Office, or my household duties, or my duties to my family. My identity was lost. I became my job and whatever else was required of me.

I felt that my purpose in life was to work and serve. It seemed to be the only things in my life that I could get half way right.

I feel like I failed in relationships and everything else.

I always wanted a mate, a husband, a companion. But it just never worked out.

Granted, I was always busy working, or going to school, or doing something for someone else that there was very little time left.

However, there were very few options presented to me. I think I may have went out on 2 or 3 dates during the 20 year span from 1996 to date. 1996 was when my last long term relationship ended. I briefly dated one man for a few months in 1999, but it also ended because it was a long distance relationship, and we just couldn't overcome that obstacle. We remained good friends until his death a few years later.

There were other male friends that I developed feelings for over the years, but they were either married or in a relationship, so that made them a "No-go" as well.

So, here I am, 43 years old, still single and childless, afflicted with an autoimmune disease with unpredictable flares of pain and fatigue, on the verge of leaving my job of 16.5 years to go on disability.

Sounds like a hot prospect, huh? I don't think so. I feel as though I am now "damaged goods". I don't want someone to feel sorry for me nor do I want to be a burden to anyone. So I feel like, who would want someone with my issues?

I generally try not to dwell on that since that would depress me to no end. I also try not to dwell on my pain, fatigue, or my disease. I have found things to keep my mind occupied during my convalescence. I do embroidery, I read, I work on this book and a few other stories when I feel the inspiration to do so, and there are some programs I watch on television. I do not sit home and watch soap operas, or reality television. I feel they are complete garbage and taint my mind.

I'm not judging those who do, they just do not interest me at all.

My health and energy has been up and down lately which is very discouraging.

I have a few decent days where I can get up and function halfway normally, only to fall down the next day and be unable to do anything.

I have been spending a lot of time completing my paperwork for my disability, whether for the retirement or my disability insurance, contacting the doctors and picking up completed paperwork and/or faxing it to the respective entities.

I have also been extremely busy with doctor's appointments. This disease requires visits to several specialists in addition to your primary doctor.

During this current term of being at home, I have seen my primary doctor, rheumatologist, endocrinologist, ophthalmologist, as well as a pulmonologist (because of chronic bronchitis and daytime fatigue they suspect sleep apnea and/or narcolepsy). I also still have an annual pap smear and mammogram that I also completed, and I had to have an eye exam with an optician to get new glasses. I am overdue for the dentist, and have no idea when I will get back there.

I have also been running to the hospital or diagnostic facility to have several tests done and have spent a night in the sleep lab recently to have a sleep study.

There are still several more appointments pending and it can be very exhausting to keep up the various doctor appointments and manage my many medications

But this is the reality of life with an autoimmune disease. I observed it for many years with my own mother, who has had lupus for over 20 years, was told about by my uncle, who has had multiple sclerosis for almost 20 years, so now it's my turn.

In spite of all the pills, paperwork, and doctor's visits, I still maintain some level of optimism. I am grateful to God for saving my life, waking me up and giving me another chance to do it right and better this time.

I was literally asleep for the last 20 years. I got up and went to work or school and fulfilled my obligations to my family, but I was not present in my life.

I know now that I often used work as an escape and was a certified workaholic.

I don't like to admit that, but I now know that it is the truth. It was the only thing I knew how to do well. Also, whenever things at home weren't going well or I had issues that I could not face or refused to face, I would throw myself into work or school so I didn't have to think about it.

Whenever overtime was needed, I did it, and I often stayed beyond my shift to complete my tasks and ensure I was caught up.

Before I knew I was ill, I would work when sick and very rarely called out. I just kept going, pushing. I was going to school, and staying up late to complete assignments and still went to work early in the morning with little or no sleep.

I would tell myself I would sleep when it was over, or when I was dead.

I gave myself a deadline to complete my studies when I was in my thirties, I announced to my family that I was to complete all matriculation by age 40 or else! I told them to beat me on the head (joking) if I fell off course.

Well the universe heard me, because I completed all requirements for my Master's degree in December 2011, when I was 39 years old and promptly submitted my application for degree. I turned 40 on January 27, 2012, and my degree arrived on my doorstep the very same day! Imagine that!

My official graduation ceremony would not take place until June 2012, but there was no joy or happiness upon completion of my studies because I was dealing with the beginning stages of this disease.

All of my future plans came to a complete halt.

I've always dreamed of working from home, working for myself, being an entrepreneur. But there was never time to do it and work too.

Maybe now I can fulfill that dream. Maybe that is why all this is happening to me.

I don't want to leave this earth without truly living and appreciating the beauty of each day.

Like Kirk Franklin says, "I had to die, so I can live!"

3/24/15

It's officially done now. I have submitted the last portion of the application for disability retirement. So now I'm just waiting for their response. Once approved, I will be able to resign/retire from the Sheriff's Office. I have also applied and have been approved for short term disability. I will continue to draw upon that until I am able to apply for social security disability.

Right now, everything is surreal. I never thought I would come to this place. I may have talked about it, wondered about it, but never imagined it would actually happen.

I'm not saying that here, wherever here is, is bad. I just felt I would be able to forge on and find a way, not realizing (until now), that I had to truly and fully surrender everything so that a change will come.

Things just could not continue the way they were. I could not go on the way that I was. So, in spite of how terrifying it feels at times, this is exactly where I need to be. As one door closes, another opens. I have left previous jobs for less.

This may be the way out the universe is providing me because I felt totally stuck, trapped, and lost. I know there are other things that I am capable of doing, other gifts that I have to share with the world, but they will remain suppressed and dormant if I remained where I was.

This illness has been a blessing, not a curse. It's not nice to be afflicted and suffer with pain and discomfort, but at least I have been given another chance at life.

It is not easy living with a disease that people cannot see. If I had a dollar for each time someone said to me, "But you don't look like there's a thing wrong with you!" I would be a rich woman.

I know that people mean well when they say that, but folks, you don't realize how much effort goes into putting myself together to function on any given day.

How much pretending and faking occurs. And makeup covers a multitude of sins, especially on a bad day.

How hard it is to go out and be around people and smile as if nothing is wrong, knowing that I'm feeling like complete and utter crap, but I refuse to complain.

And when you do attempt to explain, they just stare at you in disbelief. I can't help that you can't see when my eyes burn or my mouth hurts or my hands and feet burn or I'm exhausted or I'm achy or I'm having difficulty breathing or my joints ache.

If I could provide a visual aid, believe me I would do so. It only makes myself and others like me feel worse when we feel like we have to explain, justify, or otherwise legitimize our disease/illness/syndrome, etc.

Believe me when I tell you, that the majority of us who can no longer work, would love to go back to work if we could. It was the last thing that I wanted to do, leaving work. I did all I could to prevent it. Fought long and hard to stay.

But I was forced to go. To save myself. To maintain my sanity. To find a way for the disease to stabilize and/or go into remission. To make major and necessary lifestyle changes in my life. To find my true identity. To learn to love myself. To learn to take care of me the right way.

And this is why myself and persons like me tend to withdraw from others when dealing with our illness because we do not want to be made to feel like we are malingerers, or that this disease is all in our heads, that we are not trying hard enough, or not changing our diet, or not praying hard enough, or not going to church enough or to the right church, not taking the right medicines, not considering alternative medicine, not exercising enough, or taking vitamins, etc..

Because in spite of our best efforts, and believe you me, we have tried, at least I have, this disease still exists and has no cure. Yes, there are some with Sjogren's that have a milder form of the disease that allows them to continue to function fairly normally, continue to work full time, etc...and there are some like myself with a more aggressive form of the disease that have felt the full manifestation of symptoms and due to the debilitating nature of those symptoms and unpredictable and uncontrollable flare ups, have been forced to leave the workplace and consider or apply for some form of disability.

I still have trouble viewing myself as "disabled". I was filling out a questionnaire at the doctor's office, and when it asked for occupation, I hesitated. Since I am technically still employed, I listed my current job title, but at some point I will need to amend that to reflect my current status.

So, how do I respond to occupation now once I'm officially "retired"? Do I indicate "disabled"? Retired (though that may raise questions because of my relatively young age)? Unemployed? Homemaker?

I wonder if I will have to obtain a disabled tag for my vehicle….

I do not consider myself "disabled". If anything, my physical disability has "enabled" me to reevaluate my other abilities and explore other options and possible hidden talents.

4/25/15

No matter how long it's been since I've been dealing with all this, I'm never prepared for a flare or any unusual symptoms.

It always catches me off guard and takes a lot out of me.

I hope that no one ever thinks I or others like me would wish this upon themselves.

To have to suffer through unbearable pain and/or fatigue.

To deal with medications you don't understand and try to find one that works with minimal side effects.

To sit through endless doctors' visits and procedures.

To no longer be the active person you once were.

To have to leave work and go on some form of disability.

It is frustrating and demoralizing and your life is no longer the same.

But I know this is all happening for a reason. I just have to figure out what that is.

PEACE, QUIET, and STILLNESS

More and more I find myself finally reaching a place of peace. This is the most still I have been in my whole life. I fought this process with everything I had for as long as I could until I could fight no longer.

I don't like the way I came to be here, but I am glad that I am here. I also know that this is a temporary space that I am in because I am still evolving.

The old self is slowly leaving and I am finally allowing the new self to come in.

I had no idea that when all of this began 3 years ago that it would bring me to this point.

I had no clue that I would be forced to leave my job and start over.

I really believed I could "beat" this like I "beat" the thyroid cancer.

But what I failed to understand early on is that this needed to happen to me.

I couldn't continue going on the way that I was.

I finally realize that it's okay to not be "busy" all of the time.

And I have been spending this "quiet" time taking a long look at my life over the past 20+ years.

Too sick to work, too well to stay home

That is how I feel right now, but that's in my mind. My mind is playing tricks on me, telling me on the days I feel halfway decent that I am well enough to return to work.

But then a wave of fatigue or pain will kick in and remind me of why I have to stop working. Well, at least in an official capacity.

My feet are doing better. The swelling has decreased significantly but I still have some pain while walking.

It still has not hit me fully that I won't be returning to work.

I wouldn't call it denial but I'm in a place of suspended animation. Going through my day as usual doing what I need to do but not really giving a lot of thought to things.

But I have been appreciating the quiet and slow time. It's new and foreign to me, but I like it.

After working so hard and moving so fast for so long, it's nice to be able to take it easy.

Also, I didn't realize how tired I really was until this happened to me.

I'm really ready to just quit the job now. I'm tired of waiting and wondering.

If I just quit, then it will be over, and I can just collect my disability insurance checks while I wait on my disability retirement.

The only thing I have to figure out is how to continue my health insurance.

This is working my nerves and I don't know how much more I can take.

What does Sjogrens look like?

Is it a decrepit old woman walking bent over with a cane?

It's hard living with a disease that people can't see.

I'm sure others have seen me out socially, whether I was attending a basketball game or out to a nice dinner, or even going on a trip or two.

And knowing that I have this disease, probably wondering to themselves, "If she's so sick, how is she able to attend a sporting event, or go on a cruise?"

Then I'm sure the next thoughts are "It must be in her head, or "She must be depressed", or "Maybe she's a hypochondriac, or from the religious fanatics, "She must not be praying enough, or not living right".

Oh, and I forgot about "Maybe she's trying to get attention", or "She's just lazy and doesn't want to work". (Okay, this one anybody that knows me is the furthest thing from the truth, as hard as I've worked over the years).

All of the above are incorrect.

Like most people, people with Sjogrens or similar autoimmune diseases, we want to live a full and active life, however, our condition prevents us from doing so.

None of us wanted to stop working, if we were working, none of us wants to be confined to our homes or to our beds. None of us wants a diminished quality of life.

None of us wants or wanted to spend the rest of our days in doctor's offices, hospitals, pharmacies, and diagnostic centers.

So when we desire to go out and enjoy an activity that we previously enjoyed or to pursue a new one, we are willing to make the sacrifice to do so.

That means that we often push ourselves beyond our limits in order to accomplish certain tasks that we either need to do or want to do.

For instance, when I know that I'm going to have a busy day or want to do something that requires a lot of energy, I have to prepare myself in advance by resting a few days prior or at least making sure I take it easy just before that day arrives.

And even then there's no guarantee that that will be enough to get you through the day.

In spite of the best preparation, I have still had to cancel plans and/or appointment on the same day or the day or evening before when I see that I'm not feeling up to it.

When the day of the event or appointment arrives, I truly have to push myself and fight and pretend to get through it.

I often walk around feeling like crap or worse than crap, but still manage to paste a smile on my face.

And what people also don't know is what price is paid later for engaging in that activity the day before.

The next day or two I usually collapse from exhaustion and cannot function at all until my body has rested and recovered.

So you might see us out there attempting to live our lives as full as we can within our limitations, but don't be so quick to judge or assume we are faking or pretending illness because you cannot see the suffering we may be enduring to be able to do something we need to do or something we enjoy.

Additionally, every day is not a bad day for Sjogren's sufferers. Some days we wake up and feel great, like we were "almost" normal. So, on those days, we go out in the world with gusto! Unfortunately, those great days tend to be short lived, because at times the day begins on a high, and ends with a low!

Or, the entire day will be great, and so we go out and conduct ourselves like "normal" people, and forget we have this doggone disease! But we pay dearly for it the next day and/or the day after, and/or the day after that!

The saying, "Don't judge a book by its cover, certainly applies to Sjogren's patients!

5/6/15

Went to BSO tonight to turn in my resignation form and to say goodbye to Shelby and Tasha. I wanted to have time with both of them alone without the distractions of the office. It was appropriate because I started with both of them and had so many great memories and experiences.

It will never be goodbye though, just so long. I will continue to remain in touch with them both.

Leaving BSO is bittersweet, but necessary.

Never once did I hang my head in defeat regarding this illness. Every time I fell down, I got back up, dusted myself off, and willed myself to keep going.

If I'd had no faith, I would have and very well could have stayed flat on my back.

But I didn't.

I got up again, and again, and again.

Until I couldn't get back up anymore.

There comes a point where you have to look within yourself and be willing to ask yourself the hard questions.

<u>5/9/15</u>

Folks, please stop asking if this illness is in my mind or has to do with my state of mind.

Believe me, the type of person I am, with my work ethic and all that I've already been through, if I could will this away with my mind, I would.

I've tried the mind over matter thing, and it didn't work.

That's what often led me to push too hard.

The blood doesn't lie. What my physical body is exhibiting isn't a lie.

There is more than enough physical proof of the existence of this illness. Sometimes I feel like a person who has been falsely accused of a crime more than once, to the point where they have to carry paperwork on their person proving who they are, and that they are not the person who committed the crime.

Sometimes I feel like I need to start carrying around my lab reports and doctor's progress notes that document the levels of the Sjogren's antibodies in my blood and also show my CRP (C-Reactive Protein) levels that measure the amount of inflammation in my body and/or whether the disease is active of not.

Yeah, maybe the next time someone asks if this is in my mind, I'll just flash them with my medical paperwork.

Don't worry, I'm not angry or bitter, just thinking out loud.

If I had my way, I would have continued working.

I wish this was just in my mind, then it would be much easier to treat and cure, then I could have continued working.

I mean, all I would have needed was some antidepressants, right?

Then I would have been as good as new.

If only it was that simple.

I'm laying here now with burning eyes, a swollen foot, an aching hip, and an exhausted body.

I overdid it today and I'm paying for it.

If this feeling was in my mind, I could make it go away, but instead it lingers.

Reality and Isolation

Now that I've left the job, the reality of my disease fully hits home.

It still doesn't seem real to me that I had to leave my job of 17 years.

I'm still in the process of turning stuff in and saying goodbye, but it's over now.

I'm relieved and frightened at the same time.

I no longer have the pressure of trying to get to work when my body is telling me to stop.

But since my job was/is my identity, I feel lost without it.

However, on a positive note, I'm finally free to pursue all of the things I've ever wanted to do but never seemed to have the time.

I'm excited about that.

I feel like I've been given a chance at a new life.

I don't like the way it happened, but I understand.

I'm feeling some kind of way about how others have responded to hearing about my illness and/or my leaving the job for medical reasons.

First of all, I'm the last person who would call anyone just to complain about being sick.

I don't like to hear myself or others complain either.

We are human, and sometimes we need to vent, to get it out, to release the stress.

But no one wants to hear a sick person vent unless it's someone who has experienced the same thing or something similar, because they can truly relate.

And, sadly, I have already experienced being shunned by people I know who have distanced themselves from me once they heard I was ill.

It hurts, but I understand and still wish them well.

I know that we all have to live our lives, and I plan to do the same, so I don't expect to hear from people often, and I don't contact folks that much when I'm busy either.

I do make time to contact those I care about from time to time.

And it's nice to hear from people every now and then.

You never know when you might lifts someone's spirits with a phone call or text just to say hello.

Since I am pretty much left alone now, and no longer part of the work culture, I have withdrawn and retreated to my own little world, and slowly but surely finding some peace.

Make no mistake, I'm not sitting at home, feeling sorry for myself, and doing nothing.

Absolutely not!

I have been working on this book, as well as some other short stories based on my life experiences and trying to put the pieces of my shattered life back together.

I didn't realize what a mess my life was literally, because I was always working or going to school, and there was never any time to deal with anything.

Now I can, and when the dust has settled, I will move forward with my future plans.

Everything is new now!

I have suffered, but I can still smile.

Moving On….to the Future?

I have been wondering to myself whether my life will truly be different now.

In one sense, it already is.

It is still hard to believe that I'm finally gone from BSO.

But I know in my heart it is for the best.

All I've known for the greater part of my life is suffering, sorrow, toil, and struggle.

I have to learn how to be happy for a change and to believe that I deserve it.

I have to believe that I deserve good things and good people around me.

But it's not so easy to shed those old heavy layers of the past.

Because there's a part of me that fears that my current happiness is short-lived.

It's that old me that remains in a box, just going through the motions of life, trying to be obedient to everyone, while not honoring myself.

Now, it's time to lift myself out of the abyss, and that's more difficult than I ever imagined it would be.

I feel a little selfish at times, when I dream of my own life, my own home, my own family, my own mate.

Is this wrong?

I've been thinking deeply about this lately.

All I can do now is continue to take care of myself and look ahead to my future (albeit uncertain), with as much optimism as I can muster.

So, we have pretty much reached the end of the story, and what I have learned so far from all of this?

I need to learn to love myself, honor myself, and value myself.

It's okay to do things just for me without feeling guilty about it.

I'm worthy of love, to give love and to receive love.

I cannot give all of myself to others, all of the time.

Many of us as women, particularly black women, have been, or have had to be caretakers to our families in some way, shape or form.

We frequently put ourselves and our needs last, to ensure that everyone else's needs are taken care of. And that inherently is our nature, as women, but too many of us are paying too high a price for neglecting ourselves.

So many of us are tired.

So many of us are overworked.

So many of us are overwhelmed.

So many of us feel unappreciated.

So many of us are stressed.

So many of us feel defeated.

So many of us are depressed.

So many of us have devoted our entire lives to others.

And that is not bad in itself. We have truly shown we can be superwomen and do it all at the job, at home, at church, etc., but again, not without a price.

Too many of us as a result are suffering from hypertension.

Too many of us are having heart attacks and strokes.

Too many of us are being diagnosed with cancer.

Too many of us wake up one day old and wonder where our life went.

Too many of us are dying way too soon.

Too many of us die without having truly lived.

I had to have my entire life turned upside down and the only thing I believed I was truly good at stripped from me in order for me to realize that I was not alive, I was the living dead.

So, while it is very scary to move forward, not knowing exactly what or where I'm moving forward to, I have never felt more alive!

I appreciate and cherish every single day!

The beauty of the sunrise and sunset, lovely flowers in bloom, the serenity of the ocean, and the musical sound of children playing.

I am still dealing with the adjustment of being "retired", and of learning to rebuild my life the right way, to love myself, take care of myself, and to be fully present and alive here on earth.

Every day still presents its share of challenges and triumphs, but I am grateful to have been given another chance.

It is my sincere hope and prayer that someone is encouraged, enlightened, and inspired by my story, my experience, my journey.

We need more people to speak up and out about their experience as well.

Together we can help each other heal, cope, and educate others about Sjogren's and chronic disease!

Made in the USA
Lexington, KY
20 April 2016